The Doctor Will Be Late

Written by Dr. Sarah Carroll Smith
Illustrated by Giao Williams

PAGER PUBLICATIONS, INC.
a 501c3 non-profit literary corporation

to Patrick and Ben,
who both make waiting for the doctor entertaining

The Doctor Will Be Late

Published by Pager Publications, Inc. at pagerpublications.org.

Printed in the United States of America.

Cover design and illustrations by Giao Williams.
Book layout by Ajay Major.

First Printing: 2021

ISBN-13: 978-0-578-90128-2

A Message From The Author

The inspiration for *The Doctor Will Be Late* was conceived in many waiting rooms throughout the last several years. On multiple occasions, I found myself sitting with my children waiting for their doctors, often for an hour or more. My boys would often ask me why it took so long. They would guess reasons why the doctor was late, often surmising that she was eating candy or playing a game.

As a physician myself, I knew that this was not the case, and I would explain to them that some patients required much more time than was allowed by the schedule. I would tell them that when it was their turn, they would have the doctor's full attention. We also discussed that sometimes they may be the one with the problem or emergency that required extra time, and other people would be understanding in these circumstances.

I wrote this book to share this message, and by doing so, I hope to encourage patience and empathy in waiting rooms everywhere.

- Dr. Sarah Carroll Smith

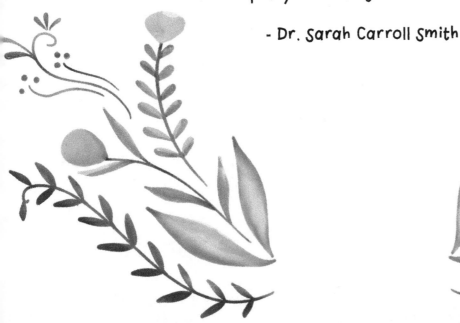
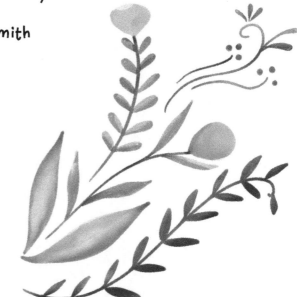

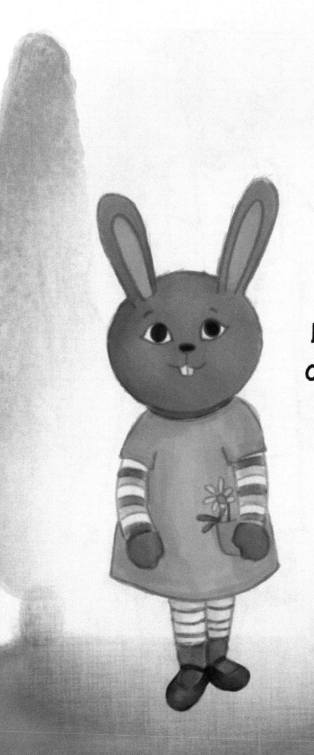

My name is
Lucy Elizabeth Brown,
and I want to tell you a
story about the best
doctor in my town.

My doctor is smart, honest, and kind.

Everyone always says, "What a wonderful doctor to find!"

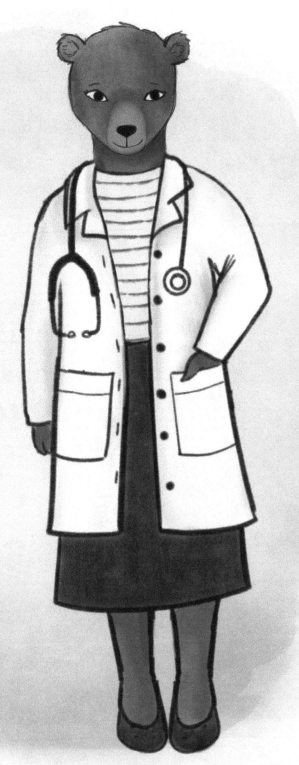

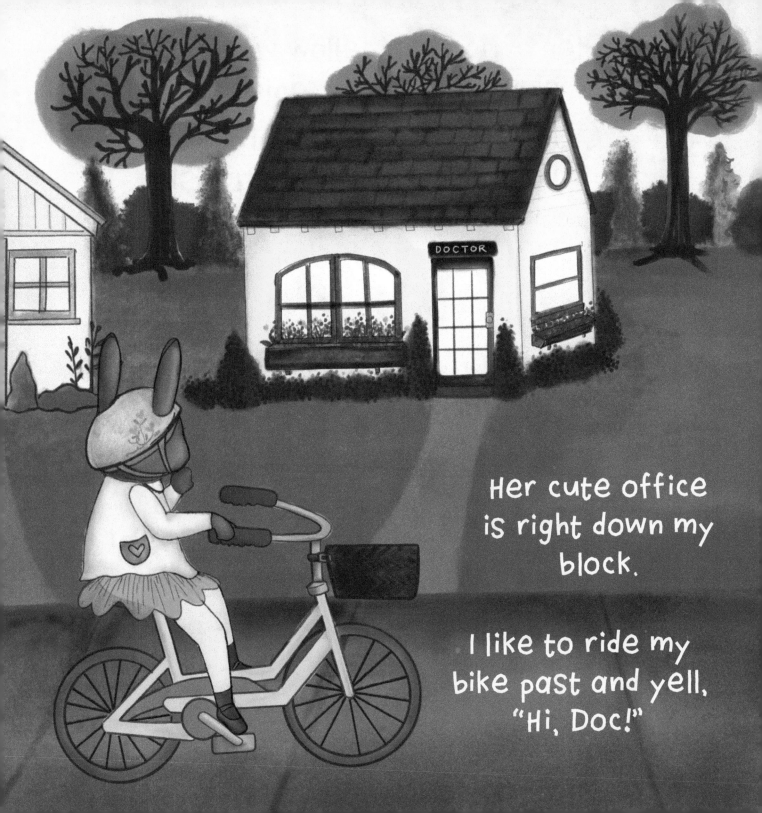

Her cute office is right down my block.

I like to ride my bike past and yell, "Hi, Doc!"

Her office has yellow walls and a
glowing tank of tropical fish.

One room even has a fountain
where you can make a wish.

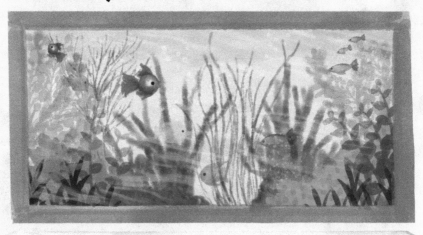

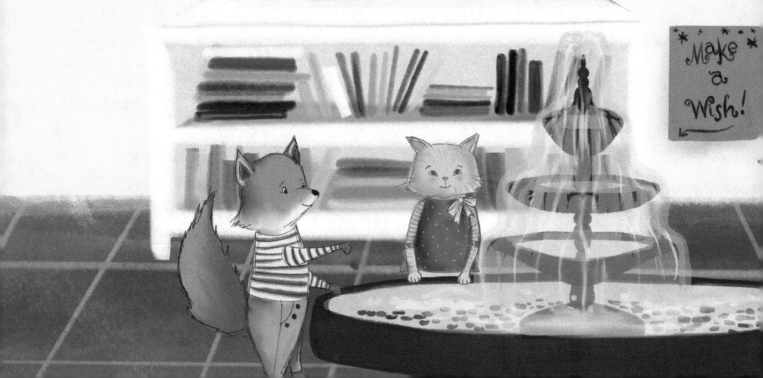

Make
a
Wish!

Doc keeps fun books scattered
around the office like loose twigs.

She sees brothers and sisters
from when they are tiny
to when they grow big.

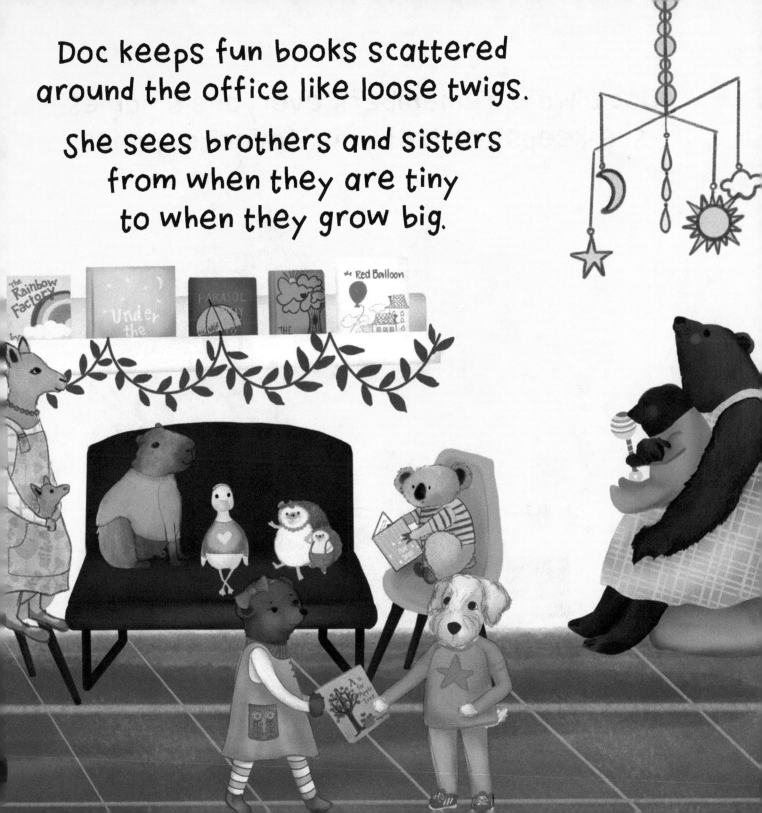

Doc always remembers everyone's names.
She keeps track of your favorite games.

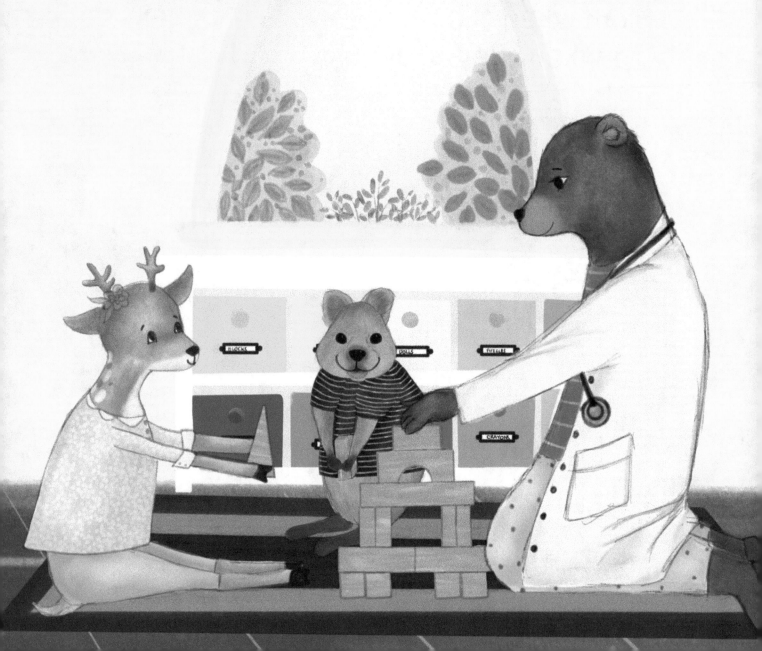

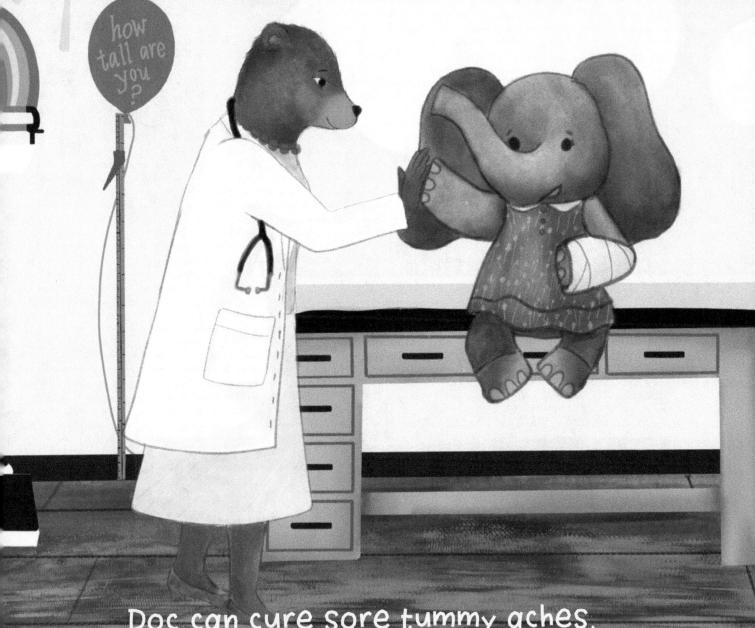

Doc can cure sore tummy aches.
She can fix a bone when it breaks.
She can stop rashes with thick, smelly creams.
Doc even likes to ask you about your crazy dreams.

Everyone loves my doctor so much. They feel better after her touch.

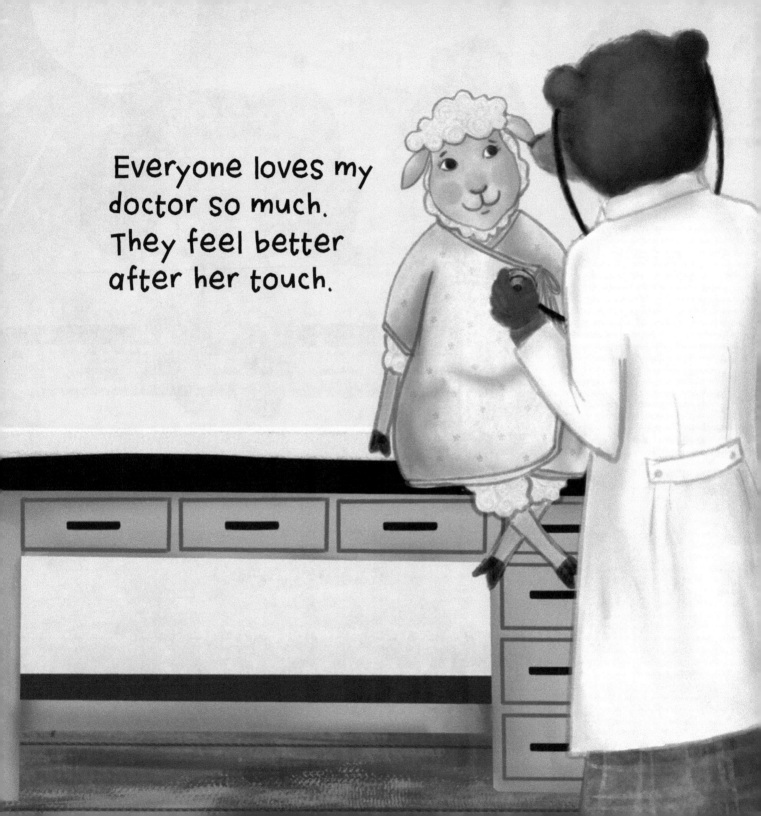

There is only one problem with visiting Doc,
and I will give you a clue...
She takes hours and hours to see everyone's crew.

When you walk in the door,
you must be prepared to
stay for many hours more.

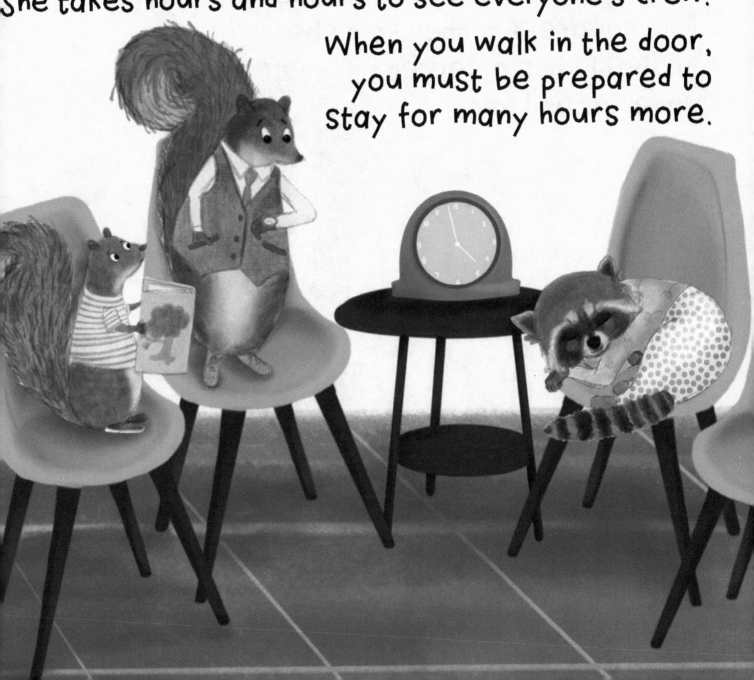

My brothers make up stories why it takes her so long. They say that Doc is eating candies and singing songs. One kid said she was playing foursquare. Another said she probably has a secret underground lair.

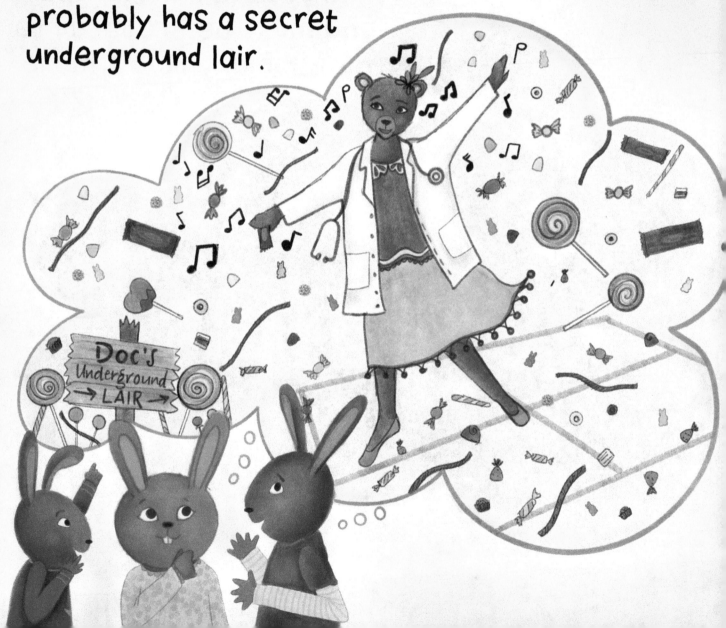

Doc's Underground → LAIR →

Everyone wonders what takes her forever.
People say they might make it out never.

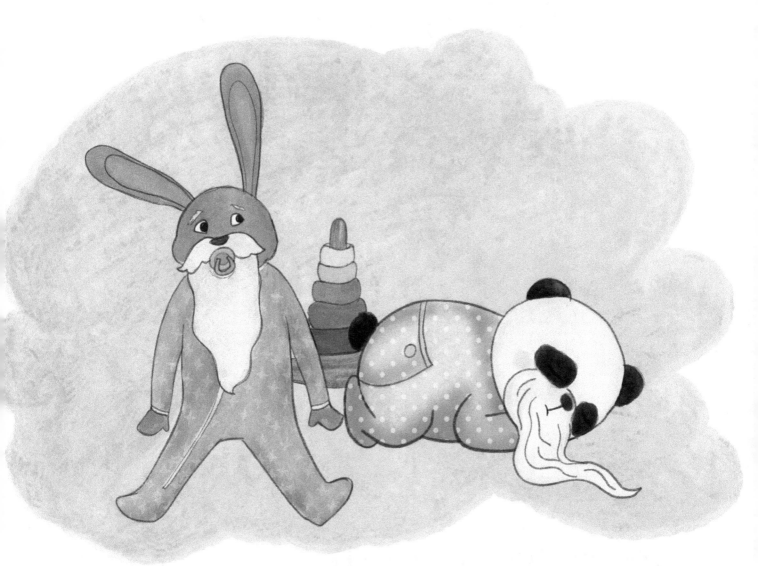

Some babies have grown old waiting.
It's a wonder she never had a bad rating.

So last time, I decided to say,
"Doc, why is there such a long wait?
How can you do it this way?"

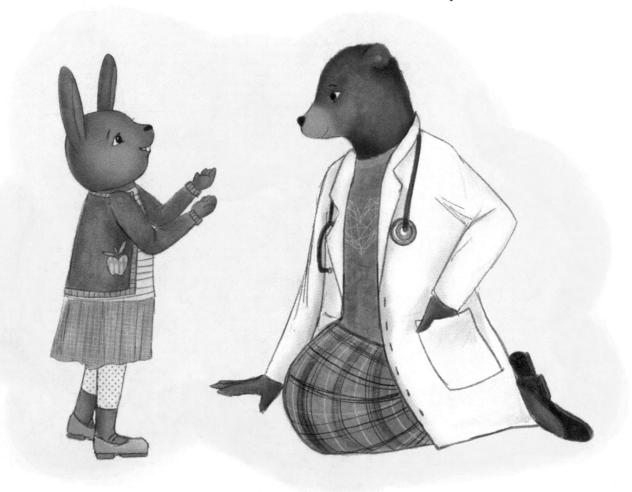

Doc got serious, and she looked in my eyes.
Everyone in the office awaited the answer
with surprise.

Then, Doc said it was because
she never wanted to turn
someone away.

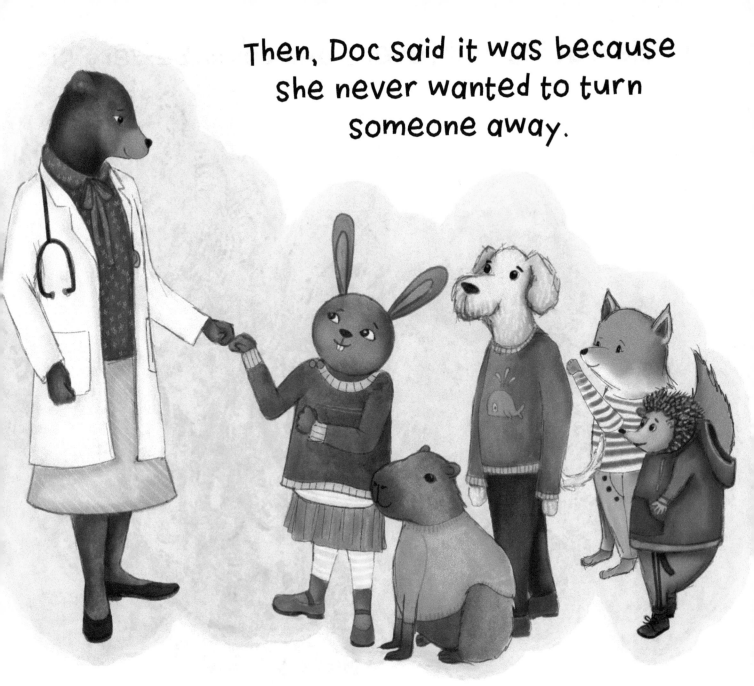

She said people needed her help,
and so she would always stay.

Little babies had fevers and could be very sick.

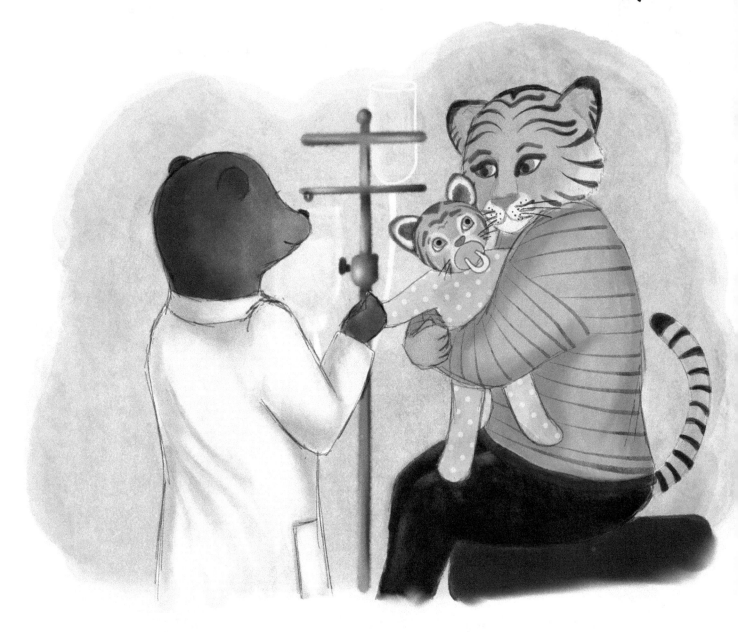

There was no way that she could be too quick.

Some kids had problems,
and they were angry or sad.

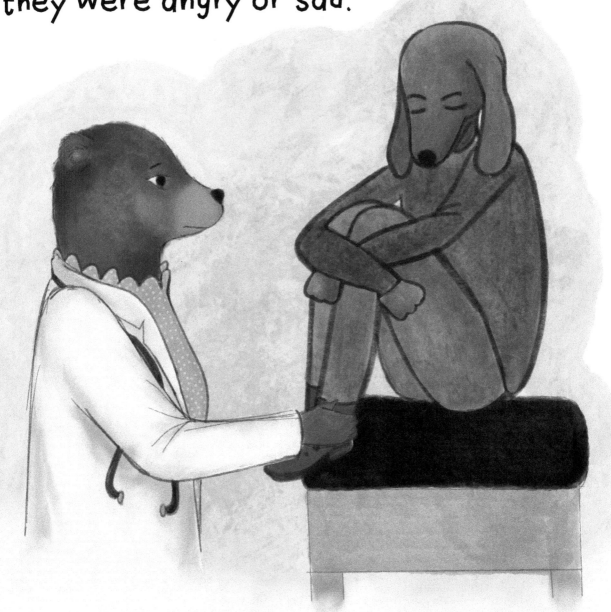

They needed extra time not to feel bad.

She said being a doctor was hard,
but she did her best.

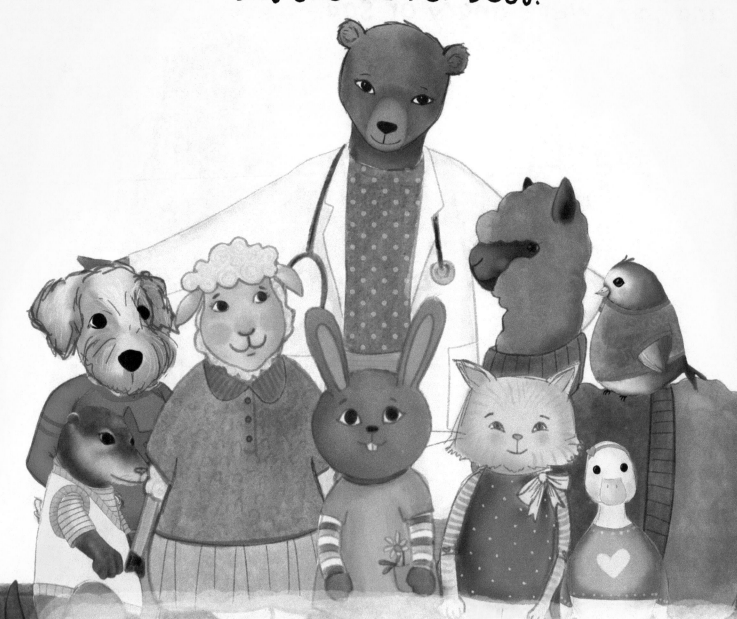

She said she loved her patients so much,
and she tried not to worry about the rest.

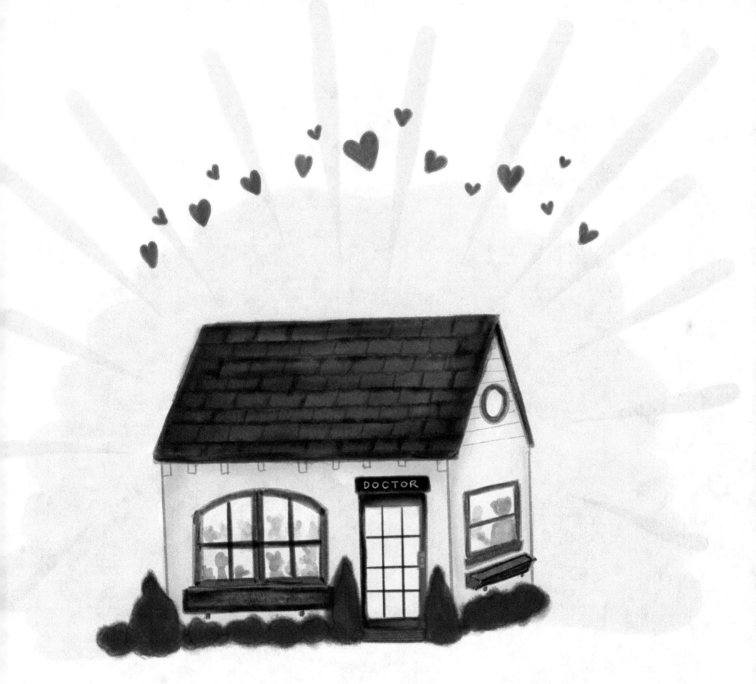

I reached up and gave Doc a hug.
I said, "Thanks! I understand now," with a shrug.

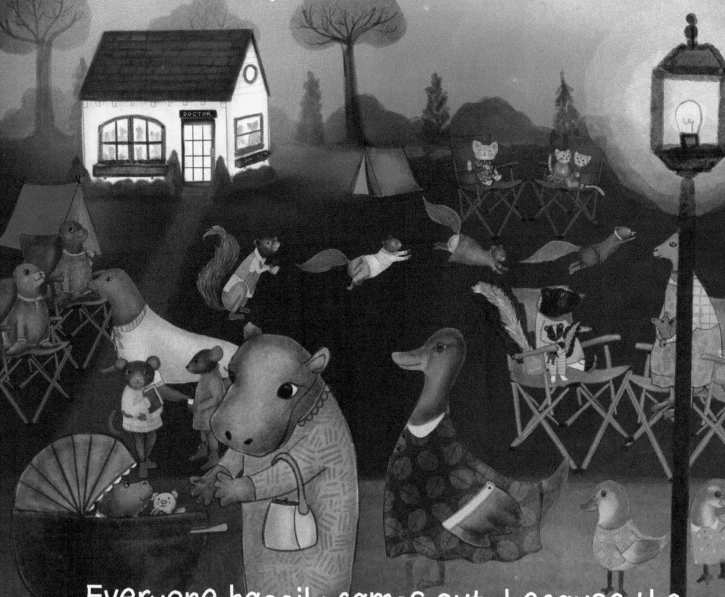

From that day on, no one complains about the wait.

Everyone happily camps out, because they understand why the doctor will be late.

Sunshine Park

Doc's Office

Farmers' Market at the Shore

Lucy's House

Lucy's town

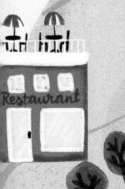
Restaurant

SCHOOL

Koala Beach

the end

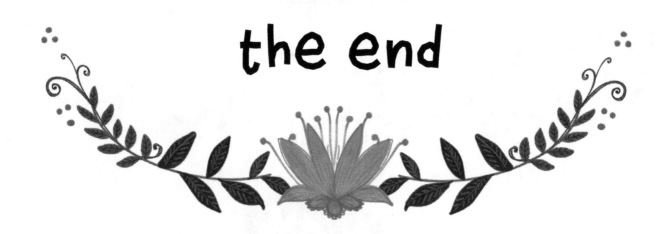

Printed in the USA
CPSIA information can be obtained
at www.ICGtesting.com
LVHW080025151123
763810LV00007B/133

9 780578 901282